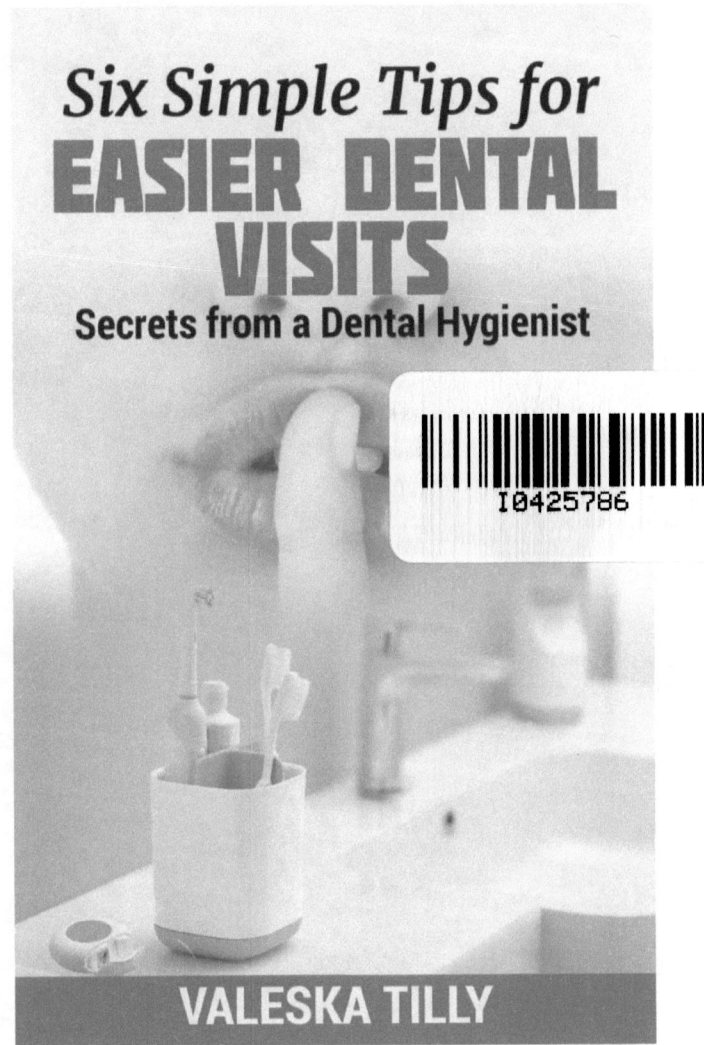

SIX SIMPLE TIPS

FOR

EASIER DENTAL VISITS:

SECRETS FROM A DENTAL HYGIENIST

———⋅⟨⟩≈⟨⟩⋅———

Valeska Tilly

Dedication

This book is dedicated to

Amelia and Tate

(who both have great teeth and gums)

With grateful thanks for being

So supportive and tolerant, and always believing in me.

With special thanks and acknowledgement to John

for his support and attention to detail

AND

to all my wonderful patients,

who listen intently to every word of advice.

May you take your teeth to heaven with you

A note from the author

This is a guide to easy dentistry at home. Six easy steps you can do at home that could help you keep your teeth for life. This book contains simple techniques from a qualified dental professional, with over 40 years' experience.

Disclaimer

The information in this book cannot be used to diagnose or treat patients. The information supplied and the opinions of the author have been simplified for general information purposes. Readers should not rely on this information as a substitute for dental diagnosis or treatment. Only you and your dentist, supported by the dental hygienist, can make appropriate dental treatment decisions about your teeth and gums.

*All the names of patients have been changed to protect their privacy.

Testimonials

As a retired dental hygienist, one of the biggest challenges in my day to day practice was empowering patients to have the confidence to carry out regular effective at home oral care. Valeska has boiled this advice down into easy-to-understand, bite-sized (pun intended) chunks of information that should be recommended reading to anyone who wants to keep their teeth for life. I wish this resource was available when I was still practicing.

Kylee Sharples,

Past President of ACT DHAA,

DHAA National Council Board Member

I read this book and found it easy to digest, logical and straight forward with a holistic approach. Anyone can easily understand and follow the advice. In my many years of dentistry I have never seen such a caring and non-judgemental approach. Well done!

Linda Greentree,

Clinical Dental Health Professional

This book is a must for anyone who wants to avoid costly procedures or loss of teeth... prevention is always better than cure, and Valeska has given clear, easy instructions on how to achieve this.

I thought I knew about gum care, and so I was surprised that I actually learnt a thing or two for my long-term gum health.

This book is not just for people with problems or concerns, but for everyone who wants to avoid them, this book is a must have for every home.

Lisa Christie,

Business Owner and Health Professional

Foreword

A very intelligent and skilled dental hygienist, Valeska has shared her extensive experience in a succinct accurate and very readable book. Valeska's advice is spot on and easy to follow.

At a time when most people want to lead a healthy lifestyle, embracing a healthy diet and exercise regime we should not overlook the health of our mouths.

The healthier your mouth is, the healthier the rest of your gut will be. The micro-biome of the bowel is topical at the moment and how improving it will have a very positive effect on the immune system and overall health.

We need to work on our mouths as well. Poor oral health is recognized as a factor in medical conditions including heart disease, diabetes and geriatric health.

Take Valeska's advice and have a long healthy and happy relationship with your mouth, improve your overall health… and take all those teeth to heaven!

Dr Susan Worboys B.D.S (Adel)

Private Practice 40 years

Duntroon Health Centre 8 years

All of those years working with wonderful Dental Hygienists including Valeska

CONTENTS

Introduction 15

1 The Birthday Cake 25

2 The Toothbrush that had Feet and The mystery 35
of the white filling that turned pink

3 The music teacher who needed to get a grip 51

4 Waking up Fresh And The Trucker 57

5 The patient who made a lifestyle change 73

6 A good relationship 79

7 Don't stop there. Keep going with your good 91
oral hygiene regime and make it a habit.

About the Author 107

SIX SIMPLE TIPS FOR EASIER DENTAL VISITS

INTRODUCTION

You want a healthy mouth, and you clean your teeth on a regular basis. Yet, you dread visits to the dentist?

Do you feel anxious when your regular dentist appointment is due?

Read on, and I will help dispel your fears.

You can be in control.

You never need to be afraid of dental visits again.

This guide will show you how, by using practical suggestions that will help boost your confidence the next time you sit in the dental chair.

Most people feel that dentistry is something that happens in a very sterile, strange environment; you lie down feeling vulnerable in a place of unusual odors, alarming looking equipment, and high-pitched noises. With a dread of discomfort, you wish it would be all over soon.

You are not alone; a lot of people don't like the experience too.

Perhaps for you it is because you are asked to hold your mouth wide open for what seems like ages.

Or allowing someone to poke and prod around inside your mouth, waiting for the verdict from the professional. Or wondering how much more discomfort you will need to endure for your treatment.

You hold your breath and tense up as you listen to the background noises and nervously await the results. Have you got decay? What is the dentist going to tell you? You sit rigid with fingers crossed, hoping that everything is good inside your mouth. Your teeth feel fine. Okay, your gums might bleed a bit every now and then, and when you floss sometimes, but nothing hurts.

The dentist delivers the verdict "To complete my examination of your mouth, I would like to take some x-rays. You may need to have three fillings. You also need to make an appointment with the hygienist for gum treatment."

WHAT?! But nothing hurts. How can this be? Do I really have three cavities? And, why do I need an appointment with the hygienist?

My gums seem fine, they don't hurt. Besides, I brush my teeth twice every day, without fail. Well, at least most of the time. Sometimes I miss brushing before bed if I've had a big night. Surely, it doesn't hurt to miss brushing once in a while?

You feel helpless and not in control of what's going on in your mouth. Your mouth's needs are being determined by someone else.

Maybe anger starts to surface, disappointment too. All you can think is; *I try my best. I brush my teeth and I buy the right toothpaste. Sure, I don't always floss, but sometimes I do. Doesn't that count for something?*

Does all this sound familiar? Do you ever think, *what else can I do?*

Do you identify with this scenario? Are you the kind of person who dreads going to the dentist every six months? Or, are you calm about your dental visits, and maybe even look forward to them?

Yes, there are people who do enjoy their dental visits! It's because they are confident they have all the right knowledge to look after their teeth and gums. They do what they need to do at home to keep their mouth healthy. These are people who do as much dentistry at home as they possibly can.

Dentistry at home? Is that even possible?

Well, it's not the same dentistry your qualified dentist, hygienist, or therapist can offer you. Nonetheless, it's still dentistry. It involves doing things yourself to maintain your own oral health. It's dentistry you can do every day, and it's fairly easy, once you know how. Another advantage is that it's cheap (compared to dentistry carried out in a clinic), and best of all, you are in control.

This book will give you six simple tips. Each one could help make a huge difference in the outcome of your next dental visit if you put them into action.

To help you think about the health needs of your mouth, and determine how you could benefit from dentistry at home, here is a simple quiz:

What is important to you?

- Do you want to keep your teeth for life?

- Is your smile important?

- Do you want to eat and chew with confidence anywhere, anytime?

- Do you feel you don't know enough about looking after your teeth & you could learn more?

- Is maintaining your dental health too difficult?

If you answered *"Yes"* to all or most of these questions, then this book could be of great value to you.

The first step is having a clear idea in your head about *what* you want for your mouth.

Your team of dental professionals is the best resource to discuss your treatment options and teach you *how* to keep your teeth for life.

Together with your dentist and hygienist, this book is a valuable guide because you will learn simple, easy tips and tricks that you can use at home to help improve your oral health.

Still not sure you can do dentistry at home? Read on and find out how.

So what is your own level of dental knowledge? Ask yourself, with regards to your specific dental needs, "How much do I really know?"

- Do you know how many times a day to brush your teeth for optimum benefit?

- Do you know how many times a day to floss your teeth for optimum benefit?
- Do you know the best type of toothpaste to use *for you* and how to use it?
- Do you know the best toothbrush to use *for your teeth* and how to use it?

If you answered *"Yes"* confidently to most of these questions, you are definitely on the way to becoming a WELL-INFORMED DENTAL INDIVIDUAL and you probably have a fairly healthy mouth.

Well done!

Now that you are in the thinking mood, here are a few more thought-provoking questions for you to consider:

- Do you wish you could eat whatever you like, such as apples or steak, etc.?
- How do you feel about your smile?
- Are you confident that your teeth and gums are healthy?

- Did you know that if your mouth is healthy, it helps to keep your whole body healthy?

Many people wish they had taken better care of their teeth when they were younger. I often hear people say, "I wish I knew 20 years ago what I know today. Maybe I wouldn't have so many silver fillings and gum problems."

This is true. If people had the knowledge 20 years ago, or even 10 years ago, they would have done more home dentistry. It would have helped them to have healthier mouths today. Alas, we can't go back in time, but we can focus on what we do now to impact our future dental health.

It's important to figure out what you want in terms of oral health.
Do you want to be more in control of your oral health? Or, do you prefer that the professionals take all the responsibility, and simply fix things *when* they go wrong?

Notice I said *when* and not *if* things go wrong, in your mouth? It's very rare for people to go through life rarely doing anything at home to maintain their dental health, and have no problems at all, ever. Even for those who have taken good care of their oral hygiene, potential problems are always lurking. Usually though, well-maintained mouths are more easily fixed than mouths that are poorly maintained. Issues are recognized earlier, and the treatment is often less invasive and less expensive. Good genes won't always keep your mouth safe from poor oral health, and poor oral health can be linked to other general health problems.

Some people believe they will solve all their dental problems by simply having all their teeth extracted. To replace them, they have a set of false teeth (dentures) inserted. Unfortunately, they don't realize that sometimes this "solution" simply creates a whole new set of different problems. For some people, a set of dentures *is* the best choice, but there are often other options that people just don't realize are available to them.

Dentures, or false teeth, need to fit properly so you are able to chew and enjoy food. Chewing with plastic teeth is very different to chewing with natural teeth. People who have dentures need to learn to chew their food a different way. Otherwise it can lead to embarrassing moments, and there can be quite a bit of discomfort. Most people don't like the idea of having false teeth, yet many believe it is inevitable that they end up with a set of dentures when they are elderly.

The truth is that most people can keep their own teeth throughout their entire life. With the right knowledge on how to keep your mouth healthy, and by practicing home dentistry and regular dental visits, keeping your own teeth can be a reality.

You may feel motivated about wanting to keep your teeth for life, and you can, if you know all your options.

So, if you are motivated to help yourself by trying some dentistry at home, you will be doing the best you can to improve your oral health, and the following chapters will be of great interest to you.

CHAPTER 1
THE BIRTHDAY CAKE

Dentistry at home is easier than you think; but you need to know how to go about it.

There are many reasons why removing the bacteria from your teeth and gums is the sensible thing to do twice a day. Why do we need to remove these bacteria?

Pain

Anyone who has ever suffered toothache will know the answer to this question. A healthy mouth makes for a happier person. If your mouth is uncomfortable, or you are in pain because your teeth are decayed, it's understandable that you will feel miserable.

Apart from the potential pain factor (as a reason for keeping your teeth and mouth in good shape), there are many more valid reasons for keeping your mouth healthy.

Your smile

Your smile is an important feature of your persona and most of us take ours for granted. Being able to smile with healthy teeth and gums is important in social settings. It also serves to boost your confidence. Inflamed red gums and stained, plaque-covered teeth are very unattractive features to see in a person's smile. If someone smiled at you with such conditions, you might unconsciously move away. We all like to see healthy teeth and gums smiling back at us.

A smile can say a lot about someone. Mostly, a smile conveys happiness. However, some people are ashamed to share their smile because their teeth are unsightly. For most people, stained, damaged or broken teeth are not something they want others to see. If someone has decayed, or missing teeth, or even swollen, bleeding or diseased gums, it's unlikely they will feel comfortable smiling at all.

It's a sad but inevitable consequence of poor oral health, and it sometimes leads to people declining social invitations for fear of being embarrassed by their teeth.

This affects their lives dramatically, especially if it reduces contact with their family, friends and community. Once their smile has been restored, their life tends to change. It sounds dramatic, I know, but many of my patients will confess to not attending social gatherings, and even doing their grocery shopping when they know less people will be around so they are less likely to feel uncomfortable when they speak to others. Placing their hand over their mouth when they talk or smile is a common practice and adjusting their smile so as to not show their teeth are also things patients report to me.

Thus, proper home care will help you maintain a healthy smile and hopefully avoid these sad consequences of an unhealthy mouth.

Bad breath

Do people take a step back from you when you are having a conversation? It might be because you have bad breath. There are many causes of bad breath, but the first and most common cause is the bacteria on the teeth and gums. It is the same bacteria that causes decay and gum disease, and it will also affect how your breath smells.

Most mouth washes and toothpastes will only cover the odor of bad breath for a short time, particularly if plaque bacteria remain in the mouth. Removal of the bacteria causing the bad odor is the best way to address this problem. Getting rid of bad breath is a good reason to develop a regular habit of brushing and flossing every day.

General health

It's not only smiling and your breath that is affected by poor oral health. Recent research[1] shows evidence of a direct link between the health of a person's mouth and their general health. For example, we now know there are links between gum disease and an increased incidence of heart disease, pneumonia and other diseases.[2] This is very significant as these ailments can be debilitating, and may affect a person's life dramatically. Research on this continues and it provides a greater understanding about significant links between diseases and oral health, especially as new links are still being discovered.

[1] https://www.ncbi.nlm.nih.gov/pmc/articles/PMC5508374/
[2] https://www.ncbi.nlm.nih.gov/pmc/articles/PMC5426403/

Other studies show links between pregnant women who have gum disease and a higher risk of giving birth prematurely. Also, in this case, the newborn baby will more than likely be underweight. This is a very important link, because newborn babies need every bit of help when they are born. To be disadvantaged by being premature and underweight, all because of the mother's gum disease is sad indeed. Such problems can be addressed, if only the mother had been aware of what she could have done beforehand.

Eating

Pain-free eating is something most people tend to take for granted. It's not until we suffer discomfort while chewing, and experience sensitivity when consuming hot or cold drinks, that we realize how important it is to have a healthy mouth. After an episode of toothache, followed by a subsequent visit to the dentist, we often wish we had been more diligent with cleaning our teeth and caring for our gums.

I will never forget a story I heard from a long-term patient at a routine check-up appointment.

She told me that she would do *anything* to keep her teeth. She had witnessed first-hand the suffering her mother had experienced with false teeth.

My patient, Mary*, went on to tell me the story of her mother's 70th birthday party. The whole family and loads of friends were present to celebrate the special occasion. Mary described the big build-up to the moment when the cake was brought out. It was a special cake made by her grand-daughters. Three tiers high, covered in pink frosting with a large *Happy 70th Birthday* on top, it was indeed a special cake. Everyone sang loudly, sharing the love in their hearts.

But when her mother went to blow out the candles, the worst possible thing happened. Unfortunately, she also blew her false teeth out of her mouth and yes, you guessed it; it flew straight into the birthday cake and lodged firmly in the pink frosting!

Embarrassed and devastated in front of everyone at the party, Mary's mother had to retrieve her false teeth from the cream frosting. Mortified, she quickly wiped her false teeth clean, popped them back in her mouth, and tried to laugh the whole incident off. Mary was so embarrassed for her mother that from that day onwards, she vowed she would do whatever it took to keep her own teeth for life. Mary never wanted to be in the same situation as her mother, *EVER!*

I hear many sad, embarrassing and regretful stories all the time from my patients. (Thankfully, some people manage to see the humorous side.) As a hygienist, it is very rewarding to be able to help patients avoid such embarrassing moments. Most of the time it's not a difficult task, you only need to know what to do for your mouth.

Cleaning your teeth and gums, twice a day, is important. It's important because the mouth is like a rubbish tip! It is full of all types of bacteria, both good and bad.

Unfortunately, you will never be able to remove all the bacteria from your mouth, but you **can** *disturb* the bacteria.

What I mean by *disturbing it* is to interrupt the tiny microorganisms from maturing and getting themselves organized.

Yes, that's right, I did say, "organized." When bacteria organize and mature (which takes around 24 hours), they start to cause serious destruction to your teeth and gums. By disturbing and cleaning away as much bacteria as you can (by brushing twice a day and flossing once a day), you have a good chance of stopping the bacteria from doing their worst to your teeth and gums.

Why twice a day?

There are a couple of reasons why dental professionals usually advise cleaning your teeth and gums twice a day. Most people lead busy lives. Many even admit that when they brush their teeth, one of the two times they brush is a rushed job. Sometimes the morning brush after breakfast is hasty, because they need to leave the house and get to work or school on time. Other people say they are too tired at night to do a good job of cleaning their mouths. This tells me that many people are brushing their teeth ineffectively at least once a day, or maybe even twice a day! Usually, this means that the bacteria removal is less efficient than it could be, and should be, to maintain good oral health. Although not enough, if there is at least one brushing a day that is thorough, this is the time when disturbing the bacteria will be most effective. Concentrate on the activity of brushing your teeth. Try not to let your mind wander. Being distracted and thinking of other things like, what will your work day involve or what will you cook for dinner that evening, takes the focus away from the job at hand. Give your teeth the time and effort they deserve. Be mindful when cleaning your teeth, do the job properly and effectively every day.

***

TIP 1:

Brush your teeth effectively twice a day.

CHAPTER 2
THE TOOTHBRUSH THAT HAD FEET
AND
THE MYSTERY OF THE WHITE FILLING
THAT TURNED PINK

It can be confusing when searching for the right toothbrush and the correct toothpaste. There are so many kinds available, and the supermarket shelves are bulging with options. It becomes overwhelming at times. On top of that, there are all the specialty brushes, flosses, in-between cleaners and rinses. There are so many to choose from that people often buy products unsuitable for their needs. They tend to buy the same brush and paste they have always bought. This results in wasting time and money, and it increases frustration. Your hygienist is the person to ask about what is right for your needs.

As a general rule, everyone should be using a toothbrush with a small head. Your brush should also be SOFT.

35

Power brush or manual brush

Whether it is a power brush or a manual brush depends on each person's needs. Some people can use a manual brush perfectly well, accomplishing good, daily plaque bacteria removal. Other people manage excellent plaque removal with a power brush. Which brush is best for you? This is a question to put to your dental professional.

As a hygienist, I can usually tell if a patient is using a power brush or a manual brush by simply looking in their mouth. Usually, their teeth are cleaner and the gums are healthier if they use a power brush. When someone switches to a power brush after using a manual one for many years, a couple of things usually happen.

It takes a little time to adjust to the power brush technique, but once it is accomplished, the patient usually feels that their mouth is cleaner. This leads to the patient being more inclined to want to be diligent with brushing, because of the noticeable improvements to their teeth and gums and the way their mouth feels. It is also easier to use a power brush. One great advantage is that plaque removal improves, leading to better oral health.

The technique for using a manual brush compared to a power brush is very different. You should ask your hygienist or dentist how to use each piece of equipment to achieve the best results.

Many people, though, do not like the feeling of a power brush. They dislike the vibrations, or the noise. I have noticed that my patients who suffer from migraine headaches often prefer not to use a power brush. Perhaps their sensitivity level is higher. Whatever the reason is for not using a power brush, there is no excuse for not using a small-sized brush. I ALWAYS recommend a small brush, manual or power.

I recall a patient of mine, Geoff*, who was "60-something" years old, did not want to use a power brush. It was difficult to get Geoff interested in all the good reasons why he should change to a power brush, AT ALL. I respected his wishes but I was emphatic that he needed to use a smaller headed toothbrush. Yet, even this suggestion was unacceptable to Geoff.

His commitment to oral hygiene was commendable; it was in fact the equipment he was using that was letting him down. I knew he was brushing his teeth on a daily basis because the areas that Geoff could reach with his adult size brush were very clean, and the gum tissue healthy. But, he was using a toothbrush that was far too large for his mouth and teeth. This caused him to inadvertently miss critical areas when brushing.

Constantly missing these areas resulted in bacterial plaque deposits all around his teeth, particularly around the last molars. I further advised him that the size of the toothbrush should be the same size as a brush for a five-year-old child.

"What!?" he exclaimed. "I'm not using a child's toothbrush."
I patiently continued my talk with him and explained the merits of using a smaller brush. Discussing how it is

easier to reach the very last tooth if the brush head is smaller. It is also much easier to reach the inside surface of the teeth (closest to the tongue), in the lower front area. This is an area that most people develop a build-up of tartar (dental professionals call this calculus) and is very difficult to reach. He was still not convinced that a small toothbrush would help him to improve his oral health. To help my case, I retrieved a toothbrush suitable for a five-year-old from my stash of samples. It was better to demonstrate in his mouth, how to use a smaller brush. At the same time, I continued to explain to Geoff that when you use a child's size brush, not only is the head size smaller, but sometimes the handle is smaller too. I suggested he look at the range in the supermarket, remembering to be mindful of the handle length so as not to make things too difficult. If the handle is too short, it might cause him to hold the toothbrush with only his fingertips while brushing!

Geoff, I could tell, was still skeptical. He confessed there was a difference when I had brushed his teeth with the smaller brush. He could definitely feel the bristles on his teeth, in places where he hadn't felt them before. It seemed that Geoff was slowly coming around to considering a smaller brush.

At the end of the appointment I gave Geoff a "goodie bag," as I do with ALL my patients. Of course, I had placed a small brush in there for him to take home. I wondered if Geoff would take my suggestions, and I wished him luck, saying I would see him in 6 months for another clean.

Well, 6 months passed and Geoff was back in my dental chair. He was a little bit of a cheeky fellow, and had a wry grin on his face at his appointment. After going through his regular medical history update, we proceeded to check Geoff's gums for disease, tartar and plaque deposits. I was in for a pleasant surprise. There were hardly any deposits of hard tartar and very little soft plaque. In fact, I had to look *REALLY* hard to find any plaque at all. Not only were Geoff's teeth cleaner, but more areas of his gums were healthier too, especially on the inside of his lower teeth. This stopped me in my tracks and I had to ask Geoff if he had changed anything in his brushing regime.

He grinned up at me from the chair and said, "Yes, I thought about what you said and decided to use a smaller brush. I didn't like the one you gave me but I did find one at the kid's section in the supermarket that I liked more."

"Good for you," I replied. "What was different about the one you found in the supermarket compared to the brush I gave you?"

"The one I chose was still for a five-year-old child, and with a small head. What I liked was the design of a cartoon character, and it also had feet on the end of the handle. Now I can stand my brush up on the bathroom shelf. I like that!"

I never would have thought that a simple design feature like feet at the end of a toothbrush would be such an important factor. It changed a grown man's thoughts about using the correct sized brush.

As a result of Geoff using the smaller head toothbrush, his plaque control had improved. In the past, his equipment had been letting him down. Now, he had the correct size for his mouth and was adept at using this new sized brush. His teeth were cleaner, his gums were healthier and there was less plaque and tartar for me to clean off. He doesn't need to visit the dentist every 6 months now. Geoff was able to extend his recall time for dental visits to 9 month intervals. He had improved his dentistry at home, and his reward was fewer visits to the dentist. Geoff is actually aiming for a 12 month recall check-up, and I believe he will be successful. All he needs to remember is to floss every day and he will be well on his way to an annual visit schedule.

Another patient had a similar experience regarding the use of correct size equipment to clean her teeth. I call it "*The mystery of the white filling that turned pink.*"

Having recently moved to my home city, Sharon* was a new patient at the dental clinic. It was her first visit with me, and actually her first visit with a hygienist. Her first appointment had been with our dentist for a check-up. Sharon had neglected to attend dental appointments for some years when she lived interstate.

The appointment with the dentist had gone well, with only a few things that needed to get done. One tooth in particular, needed a replacement filling. The original filling was a metal amalgam type and when Sharon smiled, it was easy to see the black colour. Sharon didn't like this and wanted her smile to be brighter and not show the dark metal filling. The dentist replaced it for her with a white resin filling. The tooth was also cracked and had the potential to cause decay problems which might start underneath the filling. After the filling was placed, Sharon was so delighted with the result that as she smiled at everyone, she pointed out her new filling saying, "Look at my lovely new white filling."

Sharon's family might have become a little tired of her enthusiasm, but she was very happy to have recovered her smile. Every day she looked at the filling in the mirror, inspecting it with pleasure. However, a couple of days after the filling had been done, she noticed it was starting to turn pink. Not the whole filing, but just close to the gum line. The pink area was about 3-4 mm in diameter. It was definitely turning pink. The rest of the tooth and filling were still white, just as they had been straight after the visit with the dentist. It was very curious that one part had started to turn pink.

A concerned Sharon was left wondering why this was happening. Was there something wrong with the filling? Was there something wrong with her tooth? She wasn't having any pain, so that was a good thing. Yet that pink area was causing Sharon some worries.

During her visit with me, Sharon pointed to the area that worried her, where the filling was changing colour. She explained that she didn't understand why this was happening.

I needed a closer look. Initially, it wasn't easy to see the pink area that Sharon had been describing. However, when I managed to get the right angle, it was obvious to me there was quite a thick layer of plaque on the tooth and it was coloured pink. I carefully removed the soft plaque with my instruments and asked Sharon a series of questions. I needed to know more about a few important aspects:

What type of brush was she using? Was it a manual or power brush? She informed me she was using a power brush. That was good.

What was she using to clean in between her teeth? Floss or in between bristle brushes? She said she was using little brushes. That was good.

These answers confused me. If Sharon had been doing all the right things, then why was this plaque still present on her tooth, and why was it PINK?

I asked Sharon more questions.

"Tell me about the little brushes you use," I queried.

"Well, they are quite small and they go between my teeth real easy, I really like them," Sharon replied.

I chose one of my sample in-between brushes and asked if the size was similar to the one she had been using.

"Oh no, mine is much smaller."
We had found the answer.

The equipment that Sharon had been using to clean in-between her teeth was not the correct size for her needs. Even though Sharon was diligent and cleaned every day without fail, the brush she was using was not effective in removing the plaque. The in-between brush was removing plaque from most of the tooth surfaces between the teeth, but not everywhere. As a result, there was still some plaque near the gum line. There was our culprit.

The remaining plaque had stained pink over time. Potentially, this could have caused other problems. The plaque may have started a decay area again, on that tooth and around the edge of the brand-new filling.

I removed the pink plaque carefully with my instruments, and it worked! The tooth returned to its original white color. Sharon was relieved and thankful that it was such an easy thing to fix. It was time to return to the discussion on the size of the in-between brush that Sharon had been using. I suggested she change the size to a larger one so it would be more effective. At that point, I experimented with a few sizes. We were both surprised that she needed quite a large brush to fit in between her teeth. When I asked Sharon how it felt when I used the larger brush, it was a pleasing reply. She said, "Much better, it actually feels like that area has now been cleaned properly." This was a great result. I gave Sharon some samples of the large size in-between brushes and advised her to try them at home.

When using any type of equipment in your mouth, it must be the right size for your needs. Sharon thought she was doing a great job but didn't realize she was inadvertently missing a significant area on her new filling and tooth. This may have been what led to more problems.

Although we had managed to figure out why there was plaque present on Sharon's tooth, we still did not know why it was pink. I mentioned this to Sharon and she thought about it for a while. Then I asked her what she had been eating lately.

Plaque is typically a whitish color, or similar to natural tooth color, which can make it difficult to see. If plaque remains on the teeth and you eat or drink something that can stain, such as curry, coffee, tea, or red wine, the plaque will sometimes stain to that color.

Was Sharon eating something pink or red? Maybe she was having a pink or red drink? Or (heaven forbid) a red lolly? "No," she replied, "none of those things, but I have been eating beetroot and berries every day."
"Oh, that's it!" I exclaimed. "The beetroot especially would stain the plaque pink. Plaque was present because you weren't reaching that area with the brush, and when you ate the beetroot it stained the plaque and turned it pink."

I was relieved that it was a simple solution to a problem that had really worried her.

Now Sharon has all the information she needs to enable her to clean in-between *all* her teeth correctly. She now knows the brushes need to fit snugly (without using force). This ensures proper cleaning between the teeth. The original size of in-between brushes she used was far too small, and therefore left plaque behind.

These days, Sharon has several sizes of in-between brushes, because not all the spaces between her teeth are the same size. This means that she needs to use several different sized brushes when she cleans her teeth. She is performing good dentistry at home, which helps to keep her teeth and gums strong and healthy.

Sharon's new white filling should last her a long time if she maintains effective cleaning at home every day.

***

TIP 2:

Size does matter. Use the correct size toothbrush for your mouth to achieve the best plaque removal

and

Use the correct size in-between cleaning equipment, whether it's floss or little brushes.

CHAPTER 3
THE MUSIC TEACHER WHO NEEDED TO GET A GRIP

Sarah* was a new patient of mine who booked an appointment for hygiene maintenance and therapy. Getting to know her was very interesting. She is an academic person and passionate about her career, teaching music and playing the violin.

I checked Sarah's teeth and gums. Whilst she was very diligent with brushing and flossing twice daily, her technique was letting her down. Sarah was using the correct equipment, a power brush with a soft, small head, but Sarah was missing the inside surface of the lower right molars (next to her tongue). This area can be difficult to reach for right-handed people. Equally so, the inside surface of the lower left molars is difficult for left-handed people.

When I suggested holding her toothbrush like a pen and in a vertical fashion to be able to reach the teeth she had been missing while cleaning, Sarah responded well. I used a demonstration toothbrush to show Sarah the correct technique. She was so keen to rectify her brushing technique that she immediately took ahold of the toothbrush and held it like a pen. "Like this?" she asked, excitedly.

"Yes," I assured her. "Tip the brush so it is vertical. This will make accessing the area of the lower molars that face the tongue, a lot easier. It will be more effective at removing plaque bacteria."

Sarah liked my "secret trick." She recognized the similarities between my technique in brushing, and her techniques in teaching the violin.

She told me that her pupils would go into "automatic" mode when playing a piece of music on the violin. They wouldn't think about holding the bow so they could use the whole length of the bow when they played. By doing this, they restricted themselves to only the top half of the bow. The way the pupils held and used the bow was a habit formed early on, in the practice or education phase of learning to play the violin.

"The same applies when brushing my teeth," Sarah announced.

I agreed. The similarities were obvious.

Sarah could identify the wrong technique when using the bow, and the inadequate technique when using the toothbrush.

She then summed up the conversation effectively by telling me, "It makes a big difference how you hold it!"

Habits can be good or bad.

First, we usually learn the correct way on how to do something, whether it is brushing our teeth or playing the violin. We need to be aware of the things we are learning, and why we need to use certain techniques. Holding the violin and toothbrush correctly are good examples. To remove plaque bacteria successfully in certain areas of your mouth, hold your toothbrush like a pen. Focus on the technique so you get it right. It goes with many techniques you must learn in life, whether brushing your teeth, or holding a musical instrument. To implement what you have learned, take action and be conscious of those changes. Holding the brush like a pen will ensure you reach the inside of the lower molars properly and remove plaque effectively.

Being a teacher and an academic, Sarah was interested in how people take in information and learn from the information. Interestingly, Sarah told me that 1 in 10 people will hear the instructions, understand them and implement them. The other 9 in 10 people will take longer to process to the "doing" part. As a teacher, or a hygienist, we will continue to repeat the instructions each time we see our patient, showing the secret tricks to those who need a little extra help.

Focus

It's not that the 9 out of 10 people are less intelligent, or unable to do the things requested of them. It's because they are not focusing and implementing the new instructions. They have got into their bad habits right from the onset. Or, they don't focus and they allow their minds to wander, thinking about other things while they are playing the violin, or brushing their teeth.

For the violinists who do not focus on the correct techniques, they may never move on to greater things and achieve high accomplishments in music. As for the tooth-brushers, they may never clean the tongue-side of their lower molars. This will result in a degree of gum disease and even decay.

It goes to show that focus and attention as you perform and implement the correct techniques are a valuable asset towards success!

Though simple, it's not always easy. For those violinists who do this, they might achieve greatness in the playing of their instrument. For the tooth-brushers who do this, they usually achieve a healthy score in the dental chair and are able to have extended time between visits. The tooth-brushers who focus are performing more effective dentistry at home.

***

TIP 3:

Hold your equipment correctly.

Use a grip so you can reach everywhere.

CHAPTER 4
WAKING UP FRESH AND THE TRUCKER

Unfortunately, no matter which brush you use, be it a small manual brush or a power brush, neither one will clean away all the bacteria from in between your teeth. Another piece of equipment is needed to clean these areas correctly.

Yes, you guessed it: FLOSS. It's the DENTAL "F" word. Here's a story from a patient that will make you say, "Awww…!" I sure did.

"In the past, I never used floss," a patient told me, one day.

I had been seeing Jen*, a lovely lady, for about four years as a dental patient. Jen always did her very best to maintain healthy teeth and gums. During one of her visits, she spontaneously started to tell me about her history with floss.

She explained, "I developed gum disease some years ago and my specialist dentist said I had to change my old habits to good flossing habits; otherwise I risk losing my teeth. I'd already lost some bone around my teeth, and had a lot of recession (shrinking of the gums) around most of my teeth. The situation in my mouth wasn't good. I'd wake up in the morning with my breath smelling so bad that it almost knocked me unconscious! It was terrible. I couldn't kiss my husband good morning until I'd gotten up and brushed my teeth.

Something had to change.

Now I floss my teeth before I go to bed EVERY night, and when I wake up I notice the difference. No bad breath! I kiss my husband and start the day in a lovely frame of mind. All this happened because I changed my bad habit and adopted a good habit of flossing nightly. I now start every day with a smile and a kiss, and end it with brushing and flossing."

Flossing is not easy to do effectively. Many people don't floss because it can be difficult, especially between the molar teeth. I often find that my male patients (and I don't mean to sound biased here) have trouble flossing. It can be because their hands are big and the floss is small and slippery. Achieving effective cleaning between molars is not always going to be an easy task to perform.

Flossing technique

Flossing itself is a technique that needs to be taught. Once learned, then practice is needed. I always teach my patients how to floss this way:

- Use a piece of floss of around 30-40 cm long.
- Wrap the ends of the floss around the **middle** finger on each hand, until you have a 5-6 cm length of floss between your hands.
- Use your thumbs and second (or pointer) fingers, to grasp the floss (like crab claws).
- Once you have a good grasp on the floss, you can change the angle of it to maneuver between teeth, reaching them all much easier.

- Slide the floss up and down the side of each tooth carefully, making sure to wrap the floss around the tooth surface.

This technique is not easy, and if done incorrectly, it will be ineffective.

I always recommend flossing once a day. Some of my patients floss more than once a day. That's great, if you have the time. It doesn't really matter *when* you floss; making it a daily habit is important for good oral health.

Opportunistic flossing

Some of my patients floss in the shower in the morning, after they have brushed their teeth. Others prefer to floss before bed. Then there are those, me included, who like to floss at lunchtime, especially after a eating a salad. You can be sure there will be something stuck in between your teeth after eating a salad, and it's usually green!

Many patients tell me that they floss whenever they can. This can mean from flossing in the car while waiting to pick their children up from school to sitting in front of the television in the evening. Of course, you need to be mindful not to offend other people who may be relaxing in the same room. You could always encourage them to floss too!

One of my patients proudly told me that he keeps his floss packet tucked down the side of the lounge cushion. That way he can easily retrieve it when he sits down to watch his favorite television shows.

Television flossing is a great technique for accomplishing a, let's face it, rather boring but necessary task. While relaxing and doing something else enjoyable at the same time, you won't even think about it. Voila! Doing two things at once; multitasking. Love it!

It doesn't matter when you floss, but do it at least once a day.

There are discussions amongst dental professionals about whether it is best to floss before you brush, or afterward.

My thoughts are that it doesn't matter. There are arguments for both suggestions.

If you floss before you brush, you will remove the bacteria between your teeth. The fluoride from the toothpaste can then reach this area without bacteria blocking the way.

If you floss after brushing, you are still removing bacteria from this hard to reach place in between your teeth, and achieving a clean mouth.

Types of floss

For those of you who are already flossing once a day, you may already use your favorite floss. There are several types and different brands of floss. It is important to use floss that you like, and a type you can manage. Not all flosses are the same.

Just some of the varieties of floss available (also known as Ribbon or Tape) include:

- Waxed.

- Un-waxed.

- Teflon-coated.

- Thick strands.

- Thin strands.

- Fluffy strands, Super Floss.

Floss is also available on a handle. There are a couple of designs for floss on a stick or handle. It can be shaped like a fork or shaped like a horse-shoe. Both are good designs if they work for you.

Some people like using floss with a handle, because it makes the task of cleaning between the teeth a lot easier. Whatever suits your needs is the correct floss for you.

The flossing technique can be straight-forward. It's best to discuss this with your hygienist or dentist, to make sure you are flossing correctly. It *is* possible to floss incorrectly. Some people can even inadvertently cause damage to their gums with an action that is too aggressive.

An alternative to flossing

If flossing is NOT working for you for whatever reason, perhaps your hands are too big or you can't get the floss past some of the teeth that have large fillings, don't despair and don't give up; there are other options to try. A favorite of mine is the interproximal brush. That's the professional name for the tiny brushes that look like small bottle brushes, or a tiny Christmas tree. Usually, each brand offers several sizes to accommodate the various sized spaces between the teeth. It is important to use the correct size of interproximal brush otherwise the cleaning action will largely be ineffective. If the brush is too small, you will not clean all the plaque off the tooth surface and will leave behind deposits of plaque bacteria. You will be wasting your time, and no-one wants to do that. Your dental professional will help you determine the best size for each area. The brush must fit snugly without being too loose in the space between the teeth. On the other hand, you should never force the brush into spaces between the teeth.

If used incorrectly, an interproximal brush can cause damage to the gum tissue and sometimes tooth enamel. As with floss, there are a great number of brands and types of interproximal brushes. Most are colour coded to show size differences. You may need to use 2 or 3 different colours and sizes to suit your teeth and mouth. A different size brush is needed for different sized gaps between your teeth. Most brands of interproximal brushes have a wire stem holding the bristles in place. There is also a brand made entirely of thermo-plastic. These plastic brushes appear to be gentler on the mouth and are also a bit smaller for those *REALLY* tight spots between your teeth. Alas, they are not usually as robust as the wire-based versions, but can be more effective in tiny spaces.

Using interproximal brushes is easy. Hold the brush with your fingers, and place it carefully between the teeth near the gum. Use it like a toothpick, with a gentle pushing and pulling motion to clear the bacteria from surfaces of the teeth that touch each other.

If you don't use floss or interproximal brushes, you are missing two surfaces on every tooth when you brush. Each tooth has five surfaces. If you miss two of them, then you are only cleaning 3/5 of the tooth. For every tooth in your mouth, that's only 60%! Clearly, that means brushing alone will only clean just over half of the tooth area. The surfaces that are touching together remain covered in plaque bacteria. The area in-between the teeth is a place where bacteria can make acid and develop toxins, which can then lead to decay and gum disease.

Most of us believe we are short of time. It's a common reason I hear from patients who tell me they haven't flossed. I will then suggest a method of "creating time" around their busy schedules for flossing. It can be done while watching television (as I mentioned before), and many other times during the day. It's a case of knowing about the patient's lifestyle and tailoring specific suggestions to suit them. "Opportunistic flossing" works well for many people because of their busy lives.

I recall another patient of mine, Trev*, who was 62 years old at the time. He had already lost a few of his teeth due to gum disease. There was still gum disease present around the rest of his teeth. As expected, he was not flossing or cleaning between his teeth. This is a **high-risk** category person who could potentially lose many teeth to gum disease.

Trev was a truck driver, a big man with big hands. It was obvious to me that floss was not going to be his favorite piece of oral health equipment. I talked to him for a while to understand his attitude towards flossing and cleaning in-between the teeth. I also had to find out if he wanted to keep his remaining teeth, and I needed to discover his commitment level towards his oral health.

I explained that flossing may be difficult for him because he had large hands and he may become frustrated. This was not an excuse to avoid flossing, but rather a reason why he may easily give up. The other option was to use in-between brushes. I showed him some interproximal brushes and demonstrated how to use them. Trev was a

big man and a bit of a "diamond in the rough." I
explained to him that there was a high risk he could lose
more teeth because of his gum disease. Furthermore, I
informed him that it was not too late to do something
about it to prevent any further loss of teeth. Crossing his
arms in a defensive motion, he declared, "Well, I ain't
flossin', and I ain't got time to use those fiddly little
brushes either!"

My reply to him was, "You are obviously a busy person,
and you have been honest with me on how you feel about
cleaning in-between your teeth."

At that point, he interrupted me, saying, "I guess that
means that I'll end up with false teeth then." He paused,
then continued, "I don't think I want that."

We were both silent for what seemed like ages, and then I
had an idea. I had already learned a great deal about his
attitude towards oral health, his lifestyle and his job. So, I
asked him if he wore a shirt with a top pocket to work,
whenever he was driving his truck.

"Yep," he replied, still with his arms crossed in front of him.

"GREAT!" I announced. "Can I ask you to try something? Make sure you have one interproximal brush of each size in your top pocket every day, at work. When you stop at a traffic signal, reach into your pocket and grab a little brush to clean one tooth. Clean two teeth if the traffic signals stay on long enough. Do this at every stop light, cleaning a different tooth each time. Try it for a month, then make another appointment and we'll see if it's worked for you."

After six weeks had passed, Trev, the truck driver, came back to see me in the clinic. I was flabbergasted! His teeth were clean, his gums were healthier, and he had a big smile on his face. He had successfully halted the damage that was being done by the bacteria, and his gums were healing. He had very little gum disease now, and had literally saved his own teeth by cleaning between them when he was at the traffic lights.

This method succeeded for the truck driver for a couple of reasons. He used equipment that suited him; something he could hold, and he managed to gain effective results. This sort of cleaning suited his lifestyle and busy working schedule. He opportunistically "snatched" moments during his busy day and took one small step at a time towards a healthy mouth. It really worked for this busy truck driver. It thrilled him to hear that his gum disease was stabilizing, and even improving.

He then asked me, "Does this mean I get to keep my own teeth?"

"More than likely!" I confirmed for him. "If you keep this up, your mouth will become even healthier." It was a very rewarding and happy appointment for the both of us.

I often think of my truck driver patient as a good example of how important it is to make sure people can manage their own oral health regime. Whether it's television flossing, or traffic signal brushing, if it works for you, then that's great. The complete turnaround from despair and disease, to hope and health, in the truck driver's case, was amazing. It was very rewarding for me to be able to encourage him to keep doing what he was doing. For him, that particular method of timing and commitment level worked well. He was succeeding, and he felt good about his efforts. We were both excited about his improved oral health. Trev has now completely converted to the little in-between brushes, and he never goes anywhere without a stash in his pocket.

He also confided in me that he noticed his breath is fresher. People no longer take a step back when he's talking to them. His smile is bigger, and he is much happier, all down to a small change in his dental habits, and a huge change in attitude. That was four years ago. He hasn't lost another tooth since.

I know some dental professionals, especially hygienists, are flossing fanatics. There are good reasons why we are so pushy, especially when it comes to cleaning in between your teeth.

We like our patients to keep their teeth for life. Cleaning in between them every day goes a long way to achieving that goal.

***

TIP 4:

Clean between your teeth once a day, either with floss, or small in-between brushes.

Choose a time that suits you.

CHAPTER 5
THE PATIENT WHO MADE
A LIFESTYLE CHANGE

Judy* had moved to live on a small acreage farm with her husband, Bill*, about a year ago. They loved the lifestyle of getting back to natural living. Commuting to the city for work on a daily basis was worth it.

Judy was keenly observant about her diet and exercise, and proactive on health and prevention of disease. This meant she was also diligent in attending her dental recall appointments. At the last visit though, Judy reported developing sensitive teeth.

"I can't eat my homemade ice-cream anymore, Valeska," she told me, in despair at this notion. "I REALLY like my ice-cream."

This problem had not occurred before, in the five years I had been seeing her. I wondered what had changed, and needed to get to the bottom of this. It was time to ask questions about Judy's tooth brushing habits. Had she changed to a medium or hard brush? A firm "NO," was the answer.

After a few minutes of chatting about Judy's lifestyle changes, I enquired about the source of water on the farm. It turned out that both Judy and Bill were now drinking tank water.

There is NO FLUORIDE in tank water.

As we chatted some more, I asked if anything else had changed since moving to the country, such as the toothpaste she was using.

"Oh, yes," Judy replied. "I switched over to herbal toothpaste because I thought it was better."

There lay the answer to the sensitivity in her teeth that Judy was experiencing. No fluoride in the drinking water, no fluoride in the toothpaste, and regular eating of homemade ice-cream (probably containing quite a bit of sugar).

Relieved to have been able to discover the cause of Judy's discomfort, I continued to talk with her about the benefits of fluoride. I also discussed the possible detrimental effects of herbal toothpastes.

Fluoride, apart from being a natural strengthening agent for tooth enamel, can also desensitize teeth. Most toothpaste brands on the market contain fluoride. It is a well-known fact, with a long history of research and evidence, that fluoride is highly beneficial in preventing dental decay. There are some toothpaste brands that have higher levels of fluoride, designed for people who are at more risk of dental decay. Judy and Bill were now in this higher risk group because they were only drinking tank water with no fluoride.

An added factor that caused her tooth sensitivity was more than likely Judy's use of herbal toothpaste. Often, these types of toothpaste do not contain any fluoride, but do contain harsh abrasives (usually sand, disguised by fancy names on the label). It is how these pastes attempt to clean any plaque and staining from the surface of the teeth. Unfortunately, this can also rub away enamel from the teeth, resulting in sensitivity and discomfort. Once the enamel is gone, that's it; you can't get it back.

I advised Judy to stop using her herbal toothpaste and immediately start using toothpaste containing a high fluoride level, which is only available at the pharmacy. I gave Judy specific instructions on how to use the toothpaste as well.

Judy was to use a small `dob' of paste, only about the size of a small pea, brush in her usual way (Judy was a very effective brusher) and then spit out only, no rinsing with water. Spitting out thoroughly and no rinsing will ensure a small smear layer of paste remains in the mouth. This acts as a mini strengthening treatment for the enamel of the teeth every time Judy brushes. A simple and highly effective technique which strengthens and desensitizes teeth easily; it's dentistry at home. Judy and Bill were not only at risk of tooth sensitivity, but also of increased decay rate.

Judy felt shocked. She thought she was doing the right thing by going back to "natural living." She was appreciative of the information I provided, and immediately drove to the pharmacy to purchase her toothpaste on her way home.

I phoned Judy about two weeks later to find out if her sensitivity had decreased.

"Oh! Yes," she informed me, happily. "I'm now eating my home-made ice-cream again, and so is Bill!"

All sorts of information that you provide can be relevant for your dental professional. When considering what products are right for your oral health, the hygienist will take many factors into account. These may include lifestyle, stress levels and medical history, to name a few. It is always advisable to assist your hygienist or dentist by providing them with all the information they ask for, even if you don't think it's relevant. This is so that your dental professionals can help you determine the best course of action that's right for you. Therefore, be open and honest.

***

TIP 5:

Use the correct toothpaste for your personal needs.

Make sure you are using the correct products to keep your teeth strong.

Everyone has different needs.

CHAPTER 6
A GOOD RELATIONSHIP

Patients often say, "My last dentist didn't tell me anything about how to look after my teeth and gums, and every time I went to the dentist, I needed to have at least one filling."

"Valeska, you are so interested in people's mouths, why is that?"

My answer is pretty straight-forward. I like to see people become healthier, and I know how easy it can be to improve oral health. It is rewarding for me as a professional, because people can relate to my advice. It makes sense to them, and they will benefit from the simple changes in their home dental regime. Once they start a new simple regime at home, improvement happens relatively quickly. The trick is *if it's working then keep doing it*...don't slacken off.

Most of the time, my suggestions are going to be really *simple*. The only slight difficulty is the learning and remembering of new dental hygiene routines. Usually everything I suggest or recommend is quite *easy* to implement.

When I see people for the first time, they usually require some treatment. This treatment needs to be completed first. For example, if there is decay in a tooth it may need to be restored by having a filling placed. Similarly, with gum disease, appointments need to be made and gum treatments completed.

This must happen before you can move on to the maintenance phase of the care plan.

The good news is that you don't need to learn everything about dental hygiene immediately. That's for your dental team to know. We are the dental nerds and have the expertise to understand exactly what your mouth requires to become healthy and stable. Not everyone is the same, so not everyone will benefit from the same suggestions. There are some things, though, which people can do at home that are universal, and will assist everyone to keep their mouth healthier.

I like to congratulate my patients when they have achieved a stable healthy mouth. They often demonstrate a good level of knowledge about dental health. I might even tell them, "You are almost a dental nerd like me!" I say this, of course, with respect and humor to encourage and support my patients. I want them to continue to learn about their own oral health and ways to improve. It really is easy! In order to learn and understand just about anything in life, it can help a great deal if you have a rapport with the person teaching or helping you. This is very true when it comes to dentistry.

Find the right dental team for you.
A trusted team of dental professionals is truly your best asset. Trusting your dental team to support you in your quest to keep your teeth healthy is important. Building a rapport with your dental professionals, and understanding each other, is of the utmost importance. This relationship will give you confidence in the advice that is offered. Now you have the ability to use the information at home, and work towards improving your own oral health.

I can't stress enough how important it is to communicate well with your whole dental team. From the moment you step in the door at the dental clinic, to the moment you leave, you are entitled to feel comfortable and relaxed (I know this is not easy!). Most importantly, good communication helps you to understand everything that is happening during your appointment. Reflecting on any recent dental visits may help you to remember the feelings you have when you go to the dental clinic. What is your anxiety level during dental visits?

- Do you avoid booking your next appointment at the end of the appointment you have just finished?

- When you are in the waiting room, do you feel nervous and worried about the outcome of the visit?

- Are you worried or concerned you will be "told off" by your dental professionals during your appointment?

-

- During your dental visit, do you feel you don't always understand everything that is happening?

- Do you leave feeling a level of confusion, and lacking the right information and treatment *for you?*

How you answered these questions is a good indicator about whether or not you dread going to the dental clinic. This is especially so if you answered "Yes" to most of them. You may even avoid, or put off dental appointments until something starts to hurt in your mouth. By the time pain occurs, your options for treatment are usually reduced, or are very limited. The cost of the treatment needed to restore your mouth will undoubtedly increase too.

Understanding what is happening to you is important, and having the knowledge about what is needed to keep your mouth healthy, is vital education. It is a key to helping you become more relaxed during your time in the dental clinic. You are allowed to ask questions when you are at the dentist!

Julie* presented to me as a new patient in rather a state of distress. She didn't really want an appointment with a dental hygienist; she just wanted all her lower teeth pulled out. *"I don't know why the dentist said I had to see you,"* she said, quite irritated.

I could tell immediately this was going to be no ordinary appointment. Julie's husband came into the clinic with her and sat in the corner of the room. I think Julie felt she needed support.

After checking her medical history, I commenced by asking Julie a few questions.

Had she seen a Dental Hygienist before?

Why did she want all her lower teeth pulled out?

And,

Did she know what this appointment was for?

Julie had never seen a Hygienist before and didn't really understand the role of a Hygienist in the dental surgery.

Julie had no idea why she was in my chair and simply stated she wanted her teeth pulled out.

I asked Julie about her upper denture, did it fit her mouth well?

Julie told me her denture fitted fairly well, although she couldn't really chew hard foods as it made her denture come loose in her mouth.

Julie had all her upper teeth removed at the age of 16 years. She was supposed to have the lower teeth out the next week but it was such a horrific experience on the first visit that she ran away and hid in order to miss the second dental appointment.

Since then, Julie had managed quite well with her lower teeth, until now. Now her teeth hurt nearly all the time. It was uncomfortable for Julie to eat and drink almost anything, and she wanted her teeth out. Julie was regretful she had run away from her appointment all those years ago. She wished she'd had her teeth out when she was 16 years old because she thought she wouldn't have this problem now.

It was easy to see Julie was upset and anxious about the state of her teeth and mouth. I proceeded to talk to Julie to try to understand why she wanted to have her teeth out.

"I understand you have sensitivity", I enquired.

"YES!" Julie exclaimed, "all my lower teeth hurt all the time."

I had read the file notes for Julie and the dentist had checked there was no obvious infection causing the sensitivity that was affecting Julie so much. The dentist had noted generalized recession of the gums and referred Julie to me for a gum check, a clean and oral hygiene instruction.

After checking Julie's gum health and making some clinical observations myself, I spoke at length to Julie about her sensitivity problem. I took my time and asked questions that would give me more information. I was then able to make suggestions for Julie to address her problem. I included her lovely husband in the conversation as well because he had to listen to Julie at

home when she complained about her teeth being
sensitive.

I explained the different causes of sensitivity and also the
ways to address the problem so we could fix it. I also
mentioned that I would like to at least *try* to help Julie
keep her lower teeth. One of the reasons for this, I
explained, was that sometimes it is more difficult to have
lower dentures fit properly compared to upper dentures.
They are more likely to become loose and uncomfortable.
An ill-fitting denture can cause ulcers and pain, which
makes eating and even speaking a very uncomfortable
experience.

Julie was also fearful of experiencing pain during the
clean I was about to carry out for her.

I took my time and carefully explained how I would clean
her teeth and that she could raise her hand at any time
and I would stop immediately. I reassured her that I
would be as gentle as I could. It was important to gain
Julie's trust in order for me to help her.

Julie's sensitivity was indeed caused by receding gums which exposed the root surface of all her lower teeth. Root surfaces can be sensitive to cold and hot foods and drinks, as well as sugary and acidic foods.

In order to help alleviate Julie's teeth sensitivity, I needed to explain why she had the sensitivity and then how to fix it. I asked Julie loads of questions, including what type of toothbrush and paste she was using. I completed a very gentle clean, removing plaque, calculus (tartar) and stains from her teeth both above and below the gum line and gave her instructions for a home regime.

Julie's home regime included switching to a SOFT brush. Julie had been using a medium hardness bristle toothbrush and this had definitely contributed to her receding gums. Julie had literally scrubbed away her gums in some areas. A soft brush and changing her brushing technique would stop the receding gums.

I also advised Julie to use high fluoride toothpaste. This would help to strengthen her exposed root surfaces and also help to desensitize them. To get the maximum benefit from the toothpaste, I suggested Julie brush her teeth and spit out only. NO RINSING with water. Julie thought this was rather odd.

"But won't there still be `bits' in my mouth?" She asked. I then instructed Julie to spit out thoroughly, which would indeed get rid of all the `bits' she was concerned about. As mentioned earlier, the positive effect of not rinsing is that a small smear layer of toothpaste would remain in her mouth. This meant the fluoride in the paste would keep working to strengthen and desensitize her teeth, especially her root surfaces. Julie would be, in effect, giving herself a strengthening treatment every time she brushed with no rinsing afterwards. Again, this is dentistry at home.

Julie had rarely cleaned in between her teeth, and only did when there was annoying "debris" lodged somewhere. Julie would often use a wooden toothpick to remove the "debris".

I advised Julie not to use a toothpick as it could easily splinter and cause damage to her gums. I instructed Julie on how to use small in-between brushes and I carefully checked between every tooth in order to determine the correct size for each space.

Along with using the in-between brushes on a daily basis, I suggested Julie load a small amount of toothpaste onto the brush when cleaning in-between each tooth. This meant the fluoride would reach difficult-to-access areas and strengthen and desensitize those areas as well.

I was mindful of not overwhelming Julie with instructions so I simply asked her to try my suggestions and I promised to call her in two weeks to check how her mouth was feeling. I wanted Julie to feel supported in her new home regime and confident in her ability to change how her mouth felt.

Julie's return visit to see me was very rewarding. All of Julie's teeth, except one, no longer had sensitivity. The one remaining sensitive tooth had a small decay hole causing occasional pain. The dentist restored this tooth with a simple filling and the sensitivity stopped.

Julie was full of thanks and praise for helping her attend to the suffering she had been experiencing with her sensitive teeth. "I wish I had known you 40 years ago when I had all my upper teeth pulled out. Maybe I could have kept them," Julie said regretfully. At least Julie was now more confident she could keep her lower teeth.

Julie's mouth is now very stable. She is a keen brusher and has no more sensitive teeth. Julie now eats and drinks comfortably and doesn't have to think about what she's eating and drinking before putting it in her mouth.

Julie's recall for dental checkups is every six months and I am very confident Julie will be able to extend this time soon. Her confidence improved dramatically, not only in herself but also in her approach towards attending the dentist. She was no longer fearful.

Julie was very happy to keep her teeth, and the bonus was less pain. It was also much cheaper to keep her teeth than to have them extracted.

Subsequently, Julie's nervous husband booked an appointment with me for the next week. He was suffering from almost the same issue and was impressed with the change and improvement Julie had experienced. Both Julie and her husband had great compliance with their homework and it provided great results for both of them.

It's really important to have a team of dental people you trust and can develop a good rapport with. You are allowed to ask questions during your appointment, and indeed this will assist you greatly towards a better understanding. However, sometimes you don't know what to ask because you don't know what you don't know! Simply expressing a concern or apprehension to the dental professional will start the conversation off and your knowledge will improve. You are entitled to know what's happening. During Julie's first appointment, I took a long time to try and understand her concerns. I also spent time explaining everything as clearly as I could for Julie. I helped her set goals and monitored her achievement. However, compliance with the home regime on Julie's part was required, along with support from me. We built rapport and trust together, and gained fabulous results. Julie kept her teeth.

***

TIP 6:

Select a dental team you can relate to.

This will make understanding your dental needs easier.

Developing a rapport with them will help improve

your level of knowledge and make dental visits easier.

CHAPTER 7
DON'T STOP THERE.
KEEP GOING WITH YOUR GOOD ORAL HYGIENE REGIME AND MAKE IT A HABIT.

Let's recap your home dentistry tips and a few other things.

As with any worthwhile venture in life, you hope to find the best information and advice available before you launch into doing something. Maintaining your dental health is no different.

Alas, many people feel they know what is best for their teeth and gums without the need for any training or even any reading, whatsoever. They listen to friends and relatives' experiences, allowing these stories to influence them. While these stories might have happened to someone else, the information may not be relevant to your own experience. Tales of woe and fear about their dental appointments are dreadful to hear. It's best not to listen to them.

In our age of information overload, there are many opportunities and places to gain knowledge. The internet is a great resource for gathering information. Beware though, not everything is valid, tested, or even correct, most especially when it comes to oral health.

There is a great deal of misleading information about teeth and gums. It often sounds like the truth, because of the way it is presented. It's always a good idea to keep learning, but choose a reputable source that you can rely on, and not unfounded, untrustworthy information.

Your best asset is a team of dental professionals. They have studied in their particular fields for years, and have a high level of training and experience. They will work for you and empower *you*.

It's still important to educate yourself, so your questions are pertinent. This will serve to give you more confidence in yourself, and in your dental team.

Most dental practices comprise of a general dentist and perhaps a hygienist or two. Finding a dentist who you can connect with is sometimes not easy. It's important to have a good rapport and communication with your dentist. This helps develop a mutual understanding. It will make it easier to understand your care plan, and how your home regime and dentistry fits into that "plan."

The dental hygienist plays an integral part in providing hygiene therapy. Hygienists are also responsible for assisting you with the maintenance of your teeth and gums and will provide you with ongoing support. With access to information on products and all the latest ideas in research in dentistry, they can provide you with suggestions and solutions.

Your dentist and hygienist may occasionally seek the advice of other specialists about your teeth and gums.

You may be recommended to attend an appointment for treatment with another specialist to make sure you have the best treatment options available.

The general practice dentist and hygienist will then work closely with the specialist. This ensures that you get the best care possible.

List of specialist areas in dentistry:

1. An orthodontist corrects your bite and straightens teeth.

2. An endodontist performs nerve therapy (root canal treatment).

3. A periodontist focuses on gum therapy, surgery, maintenance and placements of implants.

4. A prosthodontist specializes in the restoration and replacement of teeth with crowns, bridges, implants and dentures.

5. An oral pathologist deals with unusual pathology in the mouth. This could be lumps, bumps and unusual markings. They can also determine if cancer is present.

Different specialists have their own areas of expertise. Your own general dentist and hygienist are able to advise you, if and when you might need to see a specialist. All with the aim of ensuring you receive the appropriate dental treatment and advice.

Doing the best you can at home will help you when the time comes for your dental check-up. You will feel more confident when you lie back in the dental chair.

The best way to know what to do at home (dentistry at home) is to ask your dental professionals. Ask them relevant questions during your appointment. Some people will forget the advice as soon as they get home, so also ask for leaflets and good websites. That way you can learn about caring for your teeth in the comfort of your own home. You are more likely to understand it better because you will be more relaxed. Awareness of your teeth and gum health is important, but the professionals are there should you feel uncertain.

There are some simple things you can do though.

Chapter 1 discusses the need to brush twice a day. Don't rush when you brush, and pay attention and check for bleeding gums. After you brush and floss your teeth and you spit out, check if there is any blood in the sink. This is the *FIRST* sign of gum disease and probably the most important one for you to notice. Unlike tooth decay, gum disease rarely involves any pain, until it's too late. Many people who observe blood when spitting into the sink often don't think anything of it. Or, they may think they brushed too hard or flossed too vigorously. Sometimes this is the case, especially if you slipped with the floss or brush. More often than not, the cause of bleeding is gum disease, or inflamed gum tissue. The gum disease may not be everywhere in your mouth. There may be difficult areas to reach with your brush.

Chapter 2 talks about the correct size toothbrush for your mouth and to be effective with the in-between brushes. It's important to be able to access all areas of your mouth for effective cleaning and removal of bacterial plaque. Thus, the size of the brush needs to be tested in your own mouth. Your dental professional is the best person for this job. Once you have the correct size and brand, the rest is up to you.

Once a day is the recommendation, and it doesn't matter *when* you floss or clean with the in-between brushes. You can do it at a completely different time to your brushing, during a time of the day that suits you best. In fact, you don't even need to floss when you use in-between brushes.

Some of my patients brush their teeth in the morning and night, and floss their teeth at lunch time. It suits them to do their flossing at lunch time. Because of this, they are more inclined to do it and be successful with their dentistry at home. They've developed a habit that works for them. Figure out what works for you, and develop your own habit of home dentistry.

Flossing is sometimes VERY hard to accomplish between the back teeth. Putting two hands inside your mouth and using the correct technique with floss is not always easy. Holding your toothbrush and floss in the correct way as highlighted in Chapter 3 will enable you to be more effective with plaque removal, and therefore reduce the incidence of dental disease.

Many people ask me if it is necessary to floss every day. Chapter 4 highlights the need for in-between cleaning every day, but it doesn't really matter when. I recommend once a day flossing (or cleaning between teeth with small brushes). This will reduce the incidence of gum disease between the teeth, where the toothbrush cannot reach.

***

When I was a student at dental hygiene school, one of my professors was assessing the work I had completed for a patient. I had been discussing with the patient the importance of flossing on a daily basis. I wasn't having much success convincing the patient it was a worthwhile thing to do, so when I requested the professor to come to my clinic to check the work I had performed, I also mentioned our discussion about the importance of daily flossing. The patient then asked the professor, "Is it true what Valeska has been telling me? She says I have to floss my teeth every day!"

The professor replied, "No, you don't have to floss your teeth every day at all." He then paused for a while and my patient gave me a very smug look. Horrified, I wanted to crawl under the dental chair and hide! Perhaps I had not learnt my lessons in class well enough, because clearly, I had misunderstood flossing recommendations! I could have sworn they taught that flossing every day was the best practice to ensure healthy teeth and gums. I had read it in my reputable textbooks as well. Yet, here was the professor telling my patient that she didn't have to floss every day.

I was very confused. The textbooks and my lecturers had identified that brushing alone only removes about 60% - 70% of the plaque bacteria on teeth. The brush cannot physically reach between the teeth, where they touch each other. This is known in the dental world as the contact point, or interproximal area. Flossing is one of the best options to ensure that plaque removal happens between your teeth. The area in-between teeth is one of the most high-risk areas for tooth decay.

To my relief, the professor then clarified his statement about flossing. He continued, "No, you don't have to floss all your teeth every day at all…*only the ones you want to keep.*"

Well, did I heave a sigh of relief! I was correct after all. All my reading and the information the lecturers had given me, of course, was correct. The patient was very bemused. The smug look on her face soon vanished when she realized she had been the butt of a joke. I guess she learnt her lesson.

If you need further proof that flossing helps to remove bacteria, simply floss your teeth (yes all of them), roll the floss up and smell it. Not pleasant! You will smell the odour of the bacteria and "debris" (plaque) you have removed. If you don't floss, the plaque will stay in your mouth and lead to a source of bad breath. Even worse, it will then lead to possible decay and gum disease. If you do floss, many good things may happen, like reducing the dark red color of diseased gums and returning them to a healthy pink. The smell of bad breath will be reduced. You will have a better all-round smile and appearance, and a reduced incidence of tooth decay between the teeth.

Flossing once a day is a very important home dentistry treatment. If you are unsure about your flossing technique, your dentist or hygienist will be glad to show you how to improve at your next visit.

To be successful with plaque and bacteria removal with flossing, there are a number of products that can help you with home dentistry. We discussed these earlier, but I am referring to; floss handles, floss on a stick and specialist type flosses. They make it easier to reach all the hard-to-get to places. Then there are the tiny brushes that clean the same area as the floss, all helpful in home dentistry. I mentioned that you need a dental professional to help you with this, because in this case, size *DOES* matter.

Chapter 5 ascertains that some people require dental products that are especially suited to addressing their particular dental issues. In order for your dental professional to correctly diagnose and offer appropriate advice, it is necessary to provide all the information, whether you think it is relevant or not. This way the best outcome is achieved for your dental health.

In Chapter 6, the main point is to find a team of dental professionals who you can relate to well. A good rapport and level of understanding are aspects of a relationship that will help you feel more comfortable when visiting the dentist. More than likely you will also gain greater insight on how to care for your teeth and gums at home more effectively. Develop good communication with your dental professionals and you will benefit greatly.

By using the information provided in this book, and implementing the techniques, your confidence will grow. Your mouth will more than likely become healthier, and your next visit to the dentist will be easier.

You may even enjoy your dental visit. Imagine how you would feel at the end of your appointment if the dentist or hygienist told you that no further visits were needed and your next appointment will be in 12 months for an examination and hygiene maintenance. This is something many people strive to attain and prefer. You can too!

Use the tips outlined in this book, and any other suggestions that your dental professionals offer. Aim to develop good oral hygiene habits and you will be on the path to becoming a once-a-year check-up patient. Develop the good habits, do it for your own health, and reap the rewards.

I know you can do it. Good luck!

ABOUT THE AUTHOR

Valeska Tilly is dual-trained as a dental therapist and dental hygienist.

She commenced her training in 1977 in Adelaide, South Australia and her extensive experience in the dental field includes working in:

School Dental Services, including remote areas of Australia.

General Practice.

Specialist Orthodontic Practice.

Specialist Prosthodontics Practice.

Teaching Dental Assistants Certificate III.

Lecturing and Clinical Tutor for Dental Therapists and Dental Hygienists at university level.

Oral Health Talks for preschool children and their parents.

Supporting her patients in learning how to maintain good oral hygiene is her main focus and passion. Valeska strives to provide the best dental hygiene service and advice possible and encourages her patients to maintain their teeth for life.

By attending conferences in Australia and overseas, she maintains her knowledge of the latest research in oral hygiene techniques and equipment available. She happily passes this information on to her patients to provide them with the best there is in innovative oral health care.

Valeska currently works in a Specialist Prosthodontics Practice and is a member of:

The Dental Hygienist Association of ACT, DHAA

The Dental Hygienist Association of Australia, DHAA

The International Federation of Dental Hygienists, IFDH

The International Team for Implantology, ITI, (at time of publication, Valeska is one of only six hygienists in Australia, and also one of very few worldwide who are members of this professional association.)

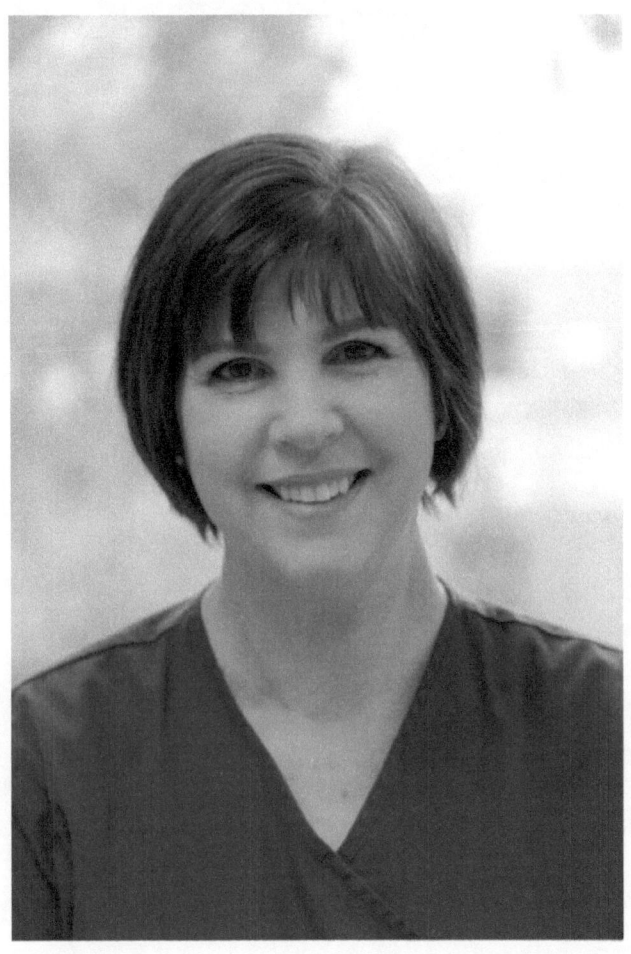

Read more about Valeska at
https://brusherbox.wixsite.com/valeskatilly.

www.ingramcontent.com/pod-product-compliance
Lightning Source LLC
Chambersburg PA
CBHW051354280526
45784CB00007B/2950